BREAKFAST AIR FRYER OVEN COOKBOOK

COOKBOOK

INSTANT VORTEX

With Love By
Catherine B. Roberts

Table Of Contents

INTRODUCTION   6

6 Reasons Why I Love Instant Vortex   **10**

GET CREATIVE   12

So Simple as... Cheese And Eggs   13

Baked Eggs In Air Fried Version   14

When I Was A Child   16

Healthy Spinach Frittata   18

Mexican Breakfast   19

Home-Fried Potatoes   21

Taste Of Home Eggs   23

   Playa Del Carmen Breakfast - Sausage And Egg Breakfast
Burrito   24

Scrambled Eggs   27

Fried Chicken And Waffles   28

Sausage In Egg Pond   30

French Toasts   33

Spinach And Bacon English Muffins   35

Yummy Potato Hash   37

Cherry Breakfast Tarts   39

Delicious Chicken Omelet   41

Omelet Frittata   43

Bacon And Hot Dogs Omelet   45

Hash Browns   46

Sausage Bacon Beans Cancan   48

Breakfast Souffle 50

Bacon And Eggs In A Cup 52

Fried Cheese Grits 54

Watermouth Toasts 56

Cheese Sandwiches 58

Tasty Zucchini Bread 60

Bacon Muffin Sandwiches 62

Nutty Banana Bread 64

Cauliflower Rice 66

Bacon Cup 68

Cheesy Tater Tot Breakfast Bake Casserole 70

Flavorful Protein Rich Breakfast 72

Breakfast Scramble Casserole 74

Egg In A Bread Basket 76

Radish Hash Browns 78

Delicious Tofu And Mushroom Omelet 80

Asparagus Frittata 82

Special Eggs, Mushroom And Tomato Scramble 84

Yummy Ham, Spinach, And Egg In A Cup 86

Mini Brown Rice Quiches 88

Glazed Strawberry Toast 90

Ham Omelet 92

Turkey Breakfast Sausage Patties 94

Tasty Cream Bread 96

Cheese Soufflés 98

CHURROS FINGERS WITH CHOCOLATE DIPPING SAUCE   100

BISCUITS DONUTS   104

A DELICIOUS FRENCH TOAST RECIPE FOR YOUR LOVER   107

Functions of Vortex Air Fryer Oven   **109**

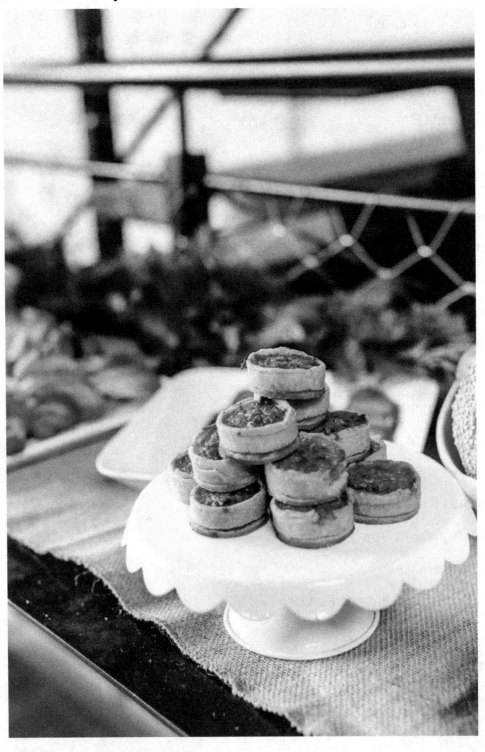

INTRODUCTION

As a mom and a food lover, I have used many different kinds of appliances for cooking. But my favorite appliance is the Instant Vortex Air Fryer Oven. You can cook different foods in it and it is very easy to use.

I don't have to spend a lot of time cooking and cleaning. I just turn on the oven and it does all the work for me.

Many people find cooking to be hard and time-consuming. They make the same recipes over and over again.

Do you find it hard to decide what to cook? You can buy a kit with all the ingredients you need, or order meat and vegetables from a restaurant. Both are easy and quick.

Restaurant food is bad for your health and it is expensive. And with meal kits, there are no opportunities to be creative.

Cooking your own food at home is a good idea because you can make the food and control what ingredients go into it.

The time you spend cooking will not be long. You can use easy recipes and the Instant Vortex so that you don't need to spend much time on it.

Breakfasts, lunch, appetizers and desserts. You can make them if you are a meat eater or vegetarian. There is something for everyone here.

The best part of these recipes is that you can make them as healthy or unhealthy as you want. You might be very hungry when reading the recipe, but don't worry.

This book is not for people who are very careful with their food. These recipes make it okay to eat some of the food you like, but if you are on a diet, there may be tips you can learn from this book.

If the diet says you can, then you can have a cheat day. You can enjoy food that is not healthy. Let's move on to see what this air fryer oven tastes like.

I enjoy cooking and creating recipes so much that I do it for a hobby.

I was thin when I was a child. Some foods I could eat without thinking of the calories. For example, onion rings, french fries, donuts and chicken fingers are fried foods.

I like these foods the most. I usually eat them when we go out to a restaurant. But now that I am getting older, I know that this is not good for me anymore.

I got fat. It was hard to lose weight. I know that you need to give up the things you love to eat. So, I ate less often at restaurants and gave away my deep-fryer in order to get more control over what I ate.

I did not enjoy my food because I could not eat what I wanted.

One day, I tried to fry things with air. I saw commercials for these machines. People always ask me if they work.

I was a little confused about the air fryer. It can cook food without all the mess. I wanted to try it anyway, but I was not sure if it would work.

I was scared to try it, but I tried it anyway. First, I tried chicken strips that were my favorite. When I tasted them they were good.

Air frying food is good because it tastes as good as food cooked with oil. It is less bad for me, and the food tastes better to me too. I like this way of cooking, so now I cook with air fryer.

After I used the Instant Vortex for a little while, I realized that it was a good way to make food. It is easy and quick. You can make small quantities of any kind of food with it.

Now that my kids are grown, they don't eat with me. I used to cook for them when they were little. Now I only cook for myself and my husband sometimes. Cooking for one or two people is really easy with the help of my Instant Vortex!

I love my air fryer. It is perfect for when I want to make a meal for myself and my husband or when friends are over.

The Instant Vortex is a machine we can use when we are camping. It helps us make food that tastes like at home even when we are camping. I love the Instant Vortex because it is easy to use and makes my favorite foods too!

All of the recipes in this book are easy to make. If you make them, they will taste good and if you have Instant Vortex, it will be even easier for you. Let's see more about it!

6 Reasons Why I Love Instant Vortex

Whether you are new to air fryers or not, this book is for you. It has recipes and tips for cooking and creativity.

If you are new to cooking, this book has many good recipes to make. More experienced cooks might find some new take on the classics that they have been making for years.

I hope you will use these recipes and love them. They can help you get a lot of good food fast.

1.Instant Vortex is good for healthy and cheap food. I can make a nutritious meal because it's fast. I don't eat out as much because Instant Vortex is healthy and cheap.

2. Instant Vortex is better for you than regular frying.

Deep fried foods have a lot of calories. There are 9 calories in each gram of fat from deep fried foods. This can make it hard to keep your calories low, but you can still eat deep fried food if you want to and make smarter choices in the rest of what you eat.

The instant vortex is magical because it makes you lose weight by reducing the number of calories you eat.

3. Instant Vortex is the best way to keep your kitchen clean. You will not need many dishes. You can put it in the air fryer and then cook it with a few bowls, so you do not need any big pots or pans.

4. The Vortex has no limits. You can make anything that you would usually cook in an oven, like appetizers like fried mozzarella sticks, to main dishes like honey baked ham, to desserts like chocolate cakes. Instant Vortex helps you make easy, healthy recipes. It is a new way to think about food that is quick and good for your body.

5. When you have All in One Appliance, you can cook with Air Fry, Broil, Bake and Reheat. There are also Rotate buttons that help for rotisserie-style cooking.

GET CREATIVE

Small kitchen appliances are helpful for us. I created every recipe in this book to save you time and money. I want your meals to be enjoyable, too.

The ingredients list is short and there are not a lot of steps to prepare the food. This book is also a source of inspiration for cooking what you like.

Instant Vortex makes cooking easy. You can change the recipes to make less food or more food, it is so versatile.

This bundle of recipes will show you how easy it is to make breakfast, side dishes, main dishes, and desserts. I am sure you will like the recipes I have made for Instant Vortex.

So Simple as... Cheese And Eggs

Serves: 2   Prep Time: 10 mins.   Cooking Time: 12 mins.

Ingredients

2-ounces of ham, sliced thinly 4 large eggs, divided

3 tablespoons of Parmesan cheese, grated finely 1/8 teaspoon of smoked paprika

2 teaspoons of fresh chives, minced 2 tablespoons of heavy cream

2 teaspoons of unsalted butter, softened Salt and black pepper, to taste

Directions

Put an egg in a bowl. Put cream and salt and pepper in the bowl too. Crack the eggs on top of the ham. Sprinkle smoked paprika, salt, and black pepper on top of everything.

Top evenly with chives and Parmesan cheese. Place the pie pan in the cooking tray. Set the Instant Vortex on Air fryer to 325 degrees F for 12 minutes.

Insert the cooking tray in the Vortex when it displays "Add Food". Remove from the oven when cooking time is complete and serve immediately.

Nutrition: Calories: 356 Protein: 24.9g Carbs: 5.4g Fat: 26.5g

Baked Eggs In Air Fried Version

Serves 2   Prep time: 5 minutes Cook time: 6 to 7 minutes

Ingredients:

2 large eggs

2 tablespoons half-and-half

2 teaspoons shredded Cheddar cheese

Salt and freshly ground black pepper, to taste
Cooking spray

Directions:

Sprinkle cooking spray on a ramekin and crack an egg into it. Pour 1 tablespoon of half-and-half and 1 teaspoon of cheese on top. Sprinkle salt and pepper too.

Stir the egg mixture with a fork until well combined. Select Bake, set temperature to 330°F (166°C), and set time to 6 minutes. Select Start to begin preheating, once preheated, place the ramekins in the oven.

When cooking is complete, the eggs should be set. Check for doneness and continue cooking for 1 minute more as needed. Allow to cool for 5 minutes before removing and serving.

Nutrition: Calories 180 Fat 18g Carbs 16g Protein 15g

When I Was A Child

Serves: 2   Prep Time: 10 mins.   Cooking Time: 15 mins.

Ingredients

1 tablespoon of olives

1 tablespoon of mustard 1 tablespoon of paprika 3 bread slices

2 tablespoons of cheddar cheese

2 eggs, whites and yolks, separated 1 tablespoon of chives

Directions

Put the bread in the tray. Turn on the Instant Vortex to 355 degrees F for 5 minutes. Put the food in when it says "Add Food".

Remove from the oven when cooking time is complete. Whisk thoroughly egg whites in a bowl and fold in the cheese, egg yolks, paprika, and mustard.

Spread this mixture over the bread slices and place in the cooking tray. Cook again in the vortex for about 10 minutes and dish out to serve.

Nutrition: Calories: 164Protein: 10.2g Carbs: 11.1g Fat: 9.2g

Healthy Spinach Frittata

Servings: 1 Preparation Time: 5 minutes Cooking Time: 8 minutes

Ingredients:

3 eggs

1 cup spinach, chopped 1 small onion, minced

2 tbsp mozzarella cheese, grated Pepper

Salt

Directions:

Preheat the air fryer to 350 F. Spray air fryer pan with cooking spray, in a bowl, whisk eggs with remaining ingredients until well combined. Pour egg mixture into the prepared pan and place pan in the air fryer basket, cook frittata for 8 minutes or until set. Serve and enjoy.

Nutrition: Calories 384 Fat 23.3 g Carbs 10.7 g Protein 34.3 g

Mexican Breakfast

Serves: 2   Prep Time: 15 mins.   Cooking Time: 8 mins.

Ingredients:

2 eggs

2 tablespoons of salsa 2 whole-wheat tortillas

4-ounces of chicken breast slices, cooked

¼ of avocado, peeled, pitted and sliced

2 tablespoons of mozzarella cheese, grated Salt and black pepper, to taste

Directions:

Mix eggs with salt and black pepper. Put egg mixture in a nonstick pan and cook for 5 minutes.

Insert the cooking tray in the Vortex when it displays "Add Food". Remove from the Vortex when cooking time is complete. Arrange the tortillas in a plate and divide the eggs, chicken slice, and avocado among the tortillas.

Top with salsa and mozzarella cheese and tightly roll each tortilla. Set the Instant Vortex on Air fryer to 355 degrees F for 3 minutes. Insert the cooking tray in the Vortex when it displays "Add Food". Remove from the oven when the tortillas become golden brown.

Nutrition: Calories: 281Protein: 26.2g Carbs: 15.4g Fat: 13g

Home-Fried Potatoes

Servings: 4   Preparation Time: 5 minutes Cooking Time: 25 minutes

Ingredients:

3 large russet potatoes 1 tablespoon canola oil

1 tablespoon extra-virgin olive oil 1 teaspoon paprika

Salt, to taste Pepper, to taste

1 cup chopped onion

1 cup chopped red bell pepper

1 cup chopped green bell pepper

Directions:

Cut the potatoes into ½-inch cubes. Place the potatoes in a large bowl of cold water and allow them to soak for at least 30 minutes, preferably an hour, dry out the potatoes and wipe thoroughly with paper towels.

Return them to the empty bowl. Add the canola and olive oils, paprika, and salt and pepper to flavor. Toss to fully coat the potatoes, transfer the potatoes to the air fryer.

Cook for 20 minutes, shaking the air fryer basket every 5 minutes (a total of 4 times). Put the onion and red and green bell peppers to the air fryer basket. Fry for an additional 3 to 4 minutes, or until the potatoes are cooked through and the peppers are soft. Cool before serving.

Nutrition: Calories 279 Fat 8g Carbs 50g Protein 6g

Taste Of Home Eggs

Serves: 2   Prep Time: 10 mins.   Cooking Time: 5 mins.

Ingredients

1 large onion, sliced
4 eggs
1/8 cup of cheddar cheese, grated
1/8 cup of mozzarella cheese, grated
¼ teaspoon of soy sauce

Directions

Cooking spray Freshly ground black pepper, to taste Whisk together eggs, black pepper, and soy sauce in a bowl. Arrange the onions in the cooking tray and top with the egg mixture and cheese. Set the Instant Vortex on Air fryer to 360 degrees F for 5 minutes. Insert the cooking tray in the Vortex when it displays "Add Food". Remove from the oven when cooking time is complete.

Serve warm.

Nutrition: Calories: 216 Protein: 15.5g Carbs: 7.9g Fat: 13.8g

Playa Del Carmen Breakfast - Sausage And Egg Breakfast Burrito

Servings: 6   Preparation Time: 5 minutes Cooking Time: 30 minutes

Ingredients:

6 eggs Salt Pepper Cooking oil

½ cup chopped red bell pepper

½ cup chopped green bell pepper 8 ounces ground chicken sausage

½ cup salsa

6 medium (8-inch) flour tortillas

½ cup shredded Cheddar cheese

Directions:

In a medium bowl, whisk the eggs. Add salt and pepper to taste, place a skillet on medium-high heat. Spray with cooking oil. Add the eggs. Scramble for 2 to 3 minutes, until the eggs are fluffy. Remove the eggs from the skillet and set aside. If needed, spray the skillet with more oil. Add the chopped red and green bell peppers. Cook for 2 to 3 minutes, once the peppers are soft, add the ground sausage to the skillet. Break the sausage into smaller pieces using a spatula or spoon. Cook for 3 to 4 minutes, until the sausage is brown, add the salsa and scrambled eggs. Stir to combine. Remove the skillet from heat. Spoon the mixture evenly onto the tortillas, to form the burritos, fold the sides of each tortilla in toward the middle and then roll up from the bottom. You can secure each burrito with a toothpick. Or you can moisten the outside edge of the tortilla with a small amount of water. I prefer to use a cooking brush, but you can also dab with your fingers. Spray the burritos with cooking oil and place them in the air fryer. Do not stack. Cook the burritos in batches if they do not all fit in the basket. Cook for 8 minutes. Open the air fryer and flip the burritos. Heat it for an additional 2 minutes or until crisp, if necessary, repeat steps 8 and 9 for the remaining burritos. Sprinkle the Cheddar cheese over the burritos. Cool before serving.

Nutrition: Calories 236 Fat 13g Carbs 16g Protein 15g

Scrambled Eggs

Serves: 2   Prep Time: 10 mins.   Cooking Time: 10 mins.

Ingredients

8 grape tomatoes, halved

½ cup of Parmesan cheese, grated ¾ cup of milk 1 tablespoon of butter

Salt and black pepper, to taste 4 eggs

Directions

Whip the eggs with milk, salt, and black pepper in a bowl. Pour the egg mixture into the cooking tray along with the grape tomatoes and cheese. Set the Instant Vortex on Air fryer to 360 degrees F for 10 minutes. Insert the cooking tray in the Vortex when it displays "Add Food". Remove from the oven when cooking time is complete. Serve warm.

Nutrition: Calories: 351Protein: 26.4g Carbs: 25.2g Fat: 22g

Fried Chicken And Waffles

Servings: 4   Preparation Time: 10 minutes Cooking Time: 30 minutes

Ingredients:

8 whole chicken wings

1 teaspoon garlic powder Chicken seasoning or rub Pepper

½ cup all-purpose flour Cooking oil

8 frozen waffles Maple syrup (optional) Directions:

In a medium bowl, spice the chicken with the garlic powder and chicken seasoning and pepper to flavor, put the chicken to a sealable plastic bag and add the flour.

Shake to thoroughly coat the chicken. Sprinkle the air fryer basket with cooking oil, with the use of tongs, put the chicken from the bag to the air fryer. It is okay to pile the chicken wings on top of each other.

Sprinkle them with cooking oil. Heat for five minutes. Unlock the air fryer and shake the basket. Presume to cook the chicken. Keep shaking every 5 minutes until 20 minutes has passed and the chicken is completely cooked, take out the cooked chicken from the air fryer and set aside.

Wash the basket and base out with warm water. Put them back to the air fryer, ease the temperature of the air fryer to 370 degrees F. Put the frozen waffles in the air fryer. Do not pile. Depends on how big your air fryer is, you may need to cook the waffles in batches. Sprinkle the waffles with cooking oil. Cook for 6 minutes, if necessary, take out the cooked waffles from the air fryer, then repeat step 9 for the leftover

 waffles. Serve the waffles with the chicken and a bit of maple syrup if desired.

Nutrition: Calories 461 Fat 22g Carbs 45g Protein 28g

Sausage In Egg Pond

Serves: 4   Prep Time: 20 mins.   Cooking Time: 20 mins.

Ingredients

1 bread slice, cut into sticks 3 eggs

2 cooked sausages, sliced

1/8 cup of Parmesan cheese, grated ¼ cup of cream 1/8 cup of mozzarella cheese, grated

Directions

Whip the eggs with cream in a bowl. Pour the egg mixture into the ramekins and fold in the sausage and bread slices. Place the ramekins in the cooking tray. Set the Instant Vortex on Air fryer to 365 degrees F for 20 minutes. Insert the cooking tray in the Vortex when it displays "Add Food". Remove from the oven when cooking time is complete. Serve warm.

Nutrition: Calories: 261 Protein: 18.3g Carbs: 4.2g Fat: 18.8g

Sausage And Cream Cheese Biscuits

Serving: 5   Preparation Time: 5 minutes Cooking Time: 15 minutes

Ingredients:

12 ounces chicken breakfast sausage 1 (6-ounce) can biscuits

⅛ cup cream cheese

Direction:

Form the sausage into 5 small patties, place the sausage patties in the air fryer. Cook for 5 minutes. Open the air fryer. Flip the patties. Cook for an additional 5 minutes, remove the cooked sausages from the air fryer. Separate the biscuit dough into 5 biscuits, place the biscuits in the air fryer. Cook for 3 minutes. Open the air fryer. Flip the biscuits. Cook for an additional 2 minutes, remove the cooked biscuits from the air fryer. Split each biscuit in half. Spread 1 teaspoon of cream cheese onto the bottom of each biscuit. Top with a sausage patty and the other half of the biscuit, and serve.

Nutrition: Calories 24g Fat 13g Carbs 20g Protein 9g

French Toasts

Serves: 2   Prep Time: 10 mins.   Cooking Time: 5 mins.

Ingredients:

2 slices of toast, whole wheat 2 oz. of salmon, smoked

4 bread slices

½ teaspoon of red chili powder ¼ cup of chickpea flour 3 tablespoons of onion, chopped finely

Water, as required

¼ teaspoon of ground turmeric

¼ teaspoon of ground cumin Salt, to taste

2 teaspoons of green chili, seeded and chopped finely

Directions:

Set the Instant Vortex on Air fryer to 375 degrees F for 4 minutes. Mingle all the ingredients in a large bowl except the bread slices. Spread this mixture over both the sides of the bread slices. Place the bread slices in the cooking tray. Insert the cooking tray in the Vortex when it displays "Add Food". Remove from the oven when cooking time is complete. Serve with tea.

Nutrition: Calories: 151   Protein: 6.5g Carbs: 26.7g   Fat: 2.3g

Spinach And Bacon English Muffins

Serves 4   Prep time: 5 minutes Cook time: 10 minutes

Ingredients:

2 strips turkey bacon, cut in half crosswise 2 whole-grain English muffins, split

1 cup fresh baby spinach, long stems removed ¼ ripe pear, peeled and thinly sliced

4 slices Provolone cheese

Directions:

Put the turkey bacon strips in a perforated pan, select Air Fry. Set temperature to 390°F (199°C) and set time to 6 minutes. Select Start to begin preheating. Once preheated, slide the pan into the oven.

Flip the strips halfway through the cooking time, when cooking is complete, the bacon should be crisp. Remove from the oven and drain on paper towels. Set aside, put the muffin halves in the perforated pan. Select Air Fry and set time to 2 minutes. Place the pan back to the oven. When done, the muffin halves will be lightly browned, remove the pan from the oven. Top each muffin half with ¼ of the baby spinach, several pear slices, a strip of turkey bacon, followed by a slice of cheese. Select Bake. Set temperature to 360°F (182°C) and set time to 2 minutes. Place the pan back to the oven.

When done, the cheese will be melted. Serve warm.

Nutrition: Calories 461 Fat 22g Carbs 45g Protein 28g

Yummy Potato Hash

Serves: 4   Prep Time: 10 mins.   Cooking Time: 40 mins.

Ingredients:

1 medium onion, chopped

½ teaspoon of thyme leaves, crushed 5 eggs, beaten

2 teaspoons of butter, melted Salt and black pepper, to taste

½ of green bell pepper, seeded and chopped 1½ pound of russet potatoes, peeled and cubed ½ teaspoon of dried savory, crushed

Directions:

Set the Instant Vortex on Air fryer to 390 degrees F for 30 minutes. Put the onion, bell pepper, thyme, potatoes, savory, salt, and black pepper in a cooking tray. Insert the cooking tray in the Vortex when it displays "Add Food". Remove from the oven when cooking time is complete. Meanwhile, add butter and whisked eggs in a skillet.

Sauté for about 1 minute on each side and place the egg pieces into the cooking tray. Cook in the vortex again for about 5 minutes and dish out to serve.

Nutrition: Calories: 229Protein: 10.3g Carbs: 30.8g Fat: 7.6g

Cherry Breakfast Tarts

Servings: 6   Preparation Time: 15 minutes Cooking Time: 20 minutes

Ingredients:

For the tarts:

2 refrigerated piecrusts

½ Cup cherry preserves 1 teaspoon cornstarch Cooking oil

For the frosting:

½ cup vanilla yogurt

1-ounce cream cheese 1 teaspoon stevia Rainbow sprinkles Directions:

To make the tarts:

Place the piecrusts on a flat surface. Make use of a knife or pizza cutter, cut each piecrust into 3 rectangles, for 6 in total. (I discard the unused dough left from slicing the edges.), in a small bowl, combine the preserves and cornstarch. Mix well. Scoop 1 tablespoon of the preserve mixture onto the top half of each piece of piecrust, fold the bottom of each piece up to close the tart. Press along the edges of each tart to seal using the back of a fork. Sprinkle the breakfast tarts with cooking oil and place them in the air fryer. I do not recommend piling the breakfast tarts. They will stick together if piled. You may need to prepare them in two batches. Cook for 10 minutes. Allow the breakfast tarts to cool fully before removing from the air fryer, if needed, repeat steps 5 and 6 for the remaining breakfast tarts.

 To make the frosting:

In a small bowl, mix the yogurt, cream cheese, and stevia. Mix well, spread the breakfast tarts with frosting and top with sprinkles, and serve.

Nutrition: Calories 119 Fat 4g Carbs 19g Protein 2g

Delicious Chicken Omelet

Serves: 8   Prep Time: 16 mins.   Cooking Time: 16 mins.

Ingredients:

½ jalapeño pepper, seeded and chopped 1 teaspoon of butter

1 onion, chopped

¼ cup of chicken, cooked and shredded Salt and black pepper, to taste

3 eggs

Directions:

Set the Instant Vortex on Air fryer to 355 degrees F for 10 minutes. Sauté onions in butter over medium heat for about 4 minutes. Stir in the chicken and jalapeño pepper. Cook for about 2 minutes and dish out in a bowl. Whip eggs with salt and black pepper in another bowl. Put the chicken mixture into the cooking tray and top with seasoned eggs. Insert the cooking tray in the Vortex when it displays "Add Food". Remove from the oven when cooking time is complete. Serve warm.

Nutrition: Calories: 209   Protein: 12g   Carbs: 11g Fat: 13g

Omelet Frittata

Servings: 2   Preparation Time: 10 minutes Cooking Time: 6 minutes

Ingredients:

3 eggs, lightly beaten

2 tbsp cheddar cheese, shredded 2 tbsp heavy cream

2 mushrooms, sliced

1/4 small onion, chopped 1/4 bell pepper, diced Pepper, to taste

Salt, to taste

Directions:

In a bowl, whisk eggs with cream, vegetables, pepper, and salt. Preheat the air fryer to 400 F. Pour egg mixture into the air fryer pan. Place pan in air fryer basket and cook for 5 minutes, add shredded cheese on top of the frittata and cook for 1 minute more. Serve and enjoy.

Nutrition: Calories 160 Fat 10 g Carbs 4 g Protein 12 g

Bacon And Hot Dogs Omelet

Serves: 2   Prep Time: 10 mins.   Cooking Time: 10 mins.

Ingredients:

2 tablespoons of milk

Salt and black pepper, to taste 4 eggs

2 hot dogs, chopped

2 small onions, chopped 1 bacon slice, chopped Directions:

Set the Instant Vortex on Air fryer to 330 degrees F for 10 minutes. Whip eggs with the remaining ingredients in a bowl. Pour the egg mixture into the cooking tray. Insert the cooking tray in the Vortex when it displays "Add Food". Remove from the oven when cooking time is complete. Serve hot.

Calories: 161   Protein: 14.1g Carbs: 5.9g   Fat: 3.4g

Hash Browns

Servings: 4   Preparation Time: 15 minutes Cooking Time: 20 minutes

Ingredients:

4 russet potatoes

1 teaspoon paprika Salt, to taste Pepper, to taste Cooking oil Directions:

Peel the potatoes using a vegetable peeler. Using a cheese grater shred the potatoes. If your grater has different-size holes, use the area of the tool with the largest holes, put the shredded potatoes in a large bowl of cold water. Let sit for 5 minutes Cold water helps remove excess starch from the potatoes. Stir to help dissolve the starch. Dry out the potatoes and dry with paper towels or napkins.

Make sure the potatoes are completely dry, Season the potatoes with the paprika and salt and pepper to taste. Spray the potatoes with cooking oil and transfer them to the air fryer. Cook for 20 minutes and shake the basket every 5 minutes (a total of 4 times). Cool before serving.

Nutrition: Calories 150 Carbs 34g Fiber 5g Protein 4g

Sausage Bacon Beans Cancan

Serves: 6   Prep Time: 10 mins.   Cooking Time: 20 mins.

Ingredients:

6 medium sausages

6 bacon slices

4 eggs

6 bread slices, toasted 1 can of baked beans

Salt and pepper, to taste

Directions:

Place the bacon and sausages in the cooking tray. Set the Instant Vortex on Air fryer to 350 degrees F for 10 minutes. Insert the cooking tray in the Vortex when it displays "Add Food". Remove from the oven when cooking time is complete. Whisk the eggs with salt and black pepper and pour in a ramekin. Put the baked beans in another ramekin. Transfer both the ramekins in the Instant Vortex and cook for about 10 minutes. Divide the sausage mixture, bread slices, eggs, and beans in serving plates to serve.

Nutrition: Calories: 518   Protein: 29.9g Carbs: 20g   Fat: 34.9g

Breakfast Souffle

Servings: 4   Preparation Time: 5 minutes Cooking Time: 15 minutes

Ingredients:

6 eggs

1/3 of cup of milk

½ cup of shredded mozzarella cheese

1 tablespoon of freshly chopped parsley

½ cup of chopped ham

1 teaspoon of black pepper

½ teaspoon of garlic powder

Directions:

Grease 4 ramekins with a nonstick cooking spray. Preheat your air fryer to 350 degrees F, using a large bowl, add and stir all the ingredients until it mixes properly. Pour the egg mixture into the greased ramekins and place it inside your air fryer, cook it inside your air fryer for 8 minutes. Then carefully remove the soufflé from your air fryer and allow it to cool off. Serve and enjoy!

Nutrition: Calories 195 Fat 15g Carbs 6g Protein 9g

Bacon And Eggs In A Cup

Serves: 2   Prep Time: 10 mins.   Cooking Time: 16 mins.

Ingredients:

2 bread slices, toasted and buttered ½ teaspoon of red pepper 1 teaspoon of marinara sauce

1 bacon slice

2 eggs

2 tablespoons of milk

1 tablespoon of Parmesan cheese, grated Freshly ground black pepper, to taste

Directions:

Place the bacon in the cooking tray. Set the Instant Vortex on Air fryer to 355 degrees F for 8 minutes. Insert the cooking tray in the Vortex when it displays "Add Food". Remove from the oven when cooking time is complete. Chop the bacon into tiny pieces and divide into 2 ramekins. Crack 1 egg in each ramekin over bacon and drizzle evenly with milk. Top with marinara sauce and Parmesan cheese.

Season with black pepper and place the ramekins in the Instant Vortex. Cook for about 8 minutes and dish out to serve.

Nutrition: Calories: 186Protein: 13.2g Carbs: 6.8g Fat: 11.7g

Fried Cheese Grits

Serves 4   Prep time: 10 minutes Cook time: 11 minutes

Ingredients:

⅔ cup instant grits

1 teaspoon salt

1 teaspoon freshly ground black pepper
¾ cup whole cream cheese

1 large egg, beaten

1 tablespoon butter, melted

1 cup shredded mild Cheddar cheese

Cooking spray

Directions:

Mix the grits, salt, and black pepper in a large bowl. Add the milk, cream cheese, beaten egg, and melted butter and whisk to combine. Fold in the Cheddar cheese and stir well, spray a baking pan with cooking spray. Spread the grits mixture into the baking pan. Select Air Fry. Set temperature to 400°F (205°C) and set time to 11 minutes. Select Start to begin preheating. Once preheated, place the pan into the oven. Stir the mixture halfway through the cooking time. When done, a knife inserted in the center should come out clean, rest for 5 minutes and serve warm.

Nutrition: Calories 150 Carbs 34g Fiber 5g Protein 4g

Watermouth Toasts

Serves: 4   Prep Time: 10 mins.   Cooking Time: 5 mins.

Ingredients:

1 cup of arugula

1 garlic clove, minced

1 teaspoon of lemon zest 4 bread slices

4-ounces of smoked salmon 1 shallot, sliced

¼ teaspoon of black pepper 8-ounces of ricotta cheese Directions:

Arrange the bread slices in the cooking tray and place in the oven. Set the Instant Vortex on Air fryer to 365 degrees F for 5 minutes. Insert the cooking tray in the Vortex when it displays "Add Food".

Remove from the oven when cooking time is complete. Process the ricotta cheese, garlic, and lemon zest in a food processor until smooth. Spread each bread slice with this mixture and top with arugula, salmon, and shallot. Serve sprinkled with black pepper.

Nutrition: Calories: 143   Protein: 12.2g Carbs: 9.2g   Fat: 6g

Cheese Sandwiches

Serves 2   Prep time: 5 minutes Cook time: 8 minutes

Ingredients:

1 teaspoon butter, softened 4 slices bread

4 slices smoked country ham 4 slices Cheddar cheese

4 thick slices tomato

Directions:

Spoon ½ teaspoon of butter onto one side of 2 slices of bread and spread it all over, assemble the sandwiches: Top each of 2 slices of unbuttered bread with 2 slices of ham, 2 slices of cheese, and 2 slices of tomato. Place the remaining 2 slices of bread on top, butter- side up.

Lay the sandwiches in a perforated pan, buttered side down, select Bake, set temperature to 370°F (188°C), and set time to 8 minutes. Select Start to begin preheating. Once preheated, slide the pan into the oven. Flip the sandwiches halfway through the cooking time. When cooking is complete, the sandwiches should be golden brown on both sides and the cheese should be melted. Remove from the oven. Allow to cool for 5 minutes before slicing to serve.

Nutrition: Calories: 186 Protein: 13.2g Carbs: 6.8g Fat: 11.7g

Tasty Zucchini Bread

Serves: 16   Prep Time: 15 mins.   Cooking Time: 20 mins.

Ingredients:

1 tablespoon of ground cinnamon 1 teaspoon of salt

2¼ cups of white sugar 1 cup of vegetable oil

3 cups of all-purpose flour 3 eggs

2 cups of zucchini, grated 1 cup of walnuts, chopped

3 teaspoons of vanilla extract

2 teaspoons of baking powder

Directions:

Strain together the baking powder, flour, cinnamon and salt in a bowl. Cream together eggs, sugar, vanilla extract and vegetable oil in another bowl. Sieve in the baking powder mixture and fold in the walnuts and zucchini.

Grease 2 loaf pans and pour this mixture into them. Place the loaf pans into the cooking tray. Set the Instant Vortex on Air fryer to 325 degrees F for 20 minutes. Insert the cooking tray in the Vortex when it displays "Add Food". Remove from the oven when cooking time is complete. Cut into preferred size slices and serve immediately.

Nutrition: Calories: 377Protein: 5.5g Carbs: 47.9g Fat: 19.3g

Bacon Muffin Sandwiches

Serves 4   Prep time: 5 minutes Cook time: 8 minutes

Ingredients:

4 English muffins, split

8 slices Canadian bacon 4 slices cheese

Cooking spray

Directions:

Make the sandwiches: Top each of 4 muffin halves with 2 slices of Canadian bacon, 1 slice of cheese, and finish with the remaining muffin half, put the sandwiches in a perforated pan and spritz the tops with cooking spray.

Select Bake, set temperature to 370°F (188°C), and set time to 8 minutes. Select Start to begin preheating, once preheated, slide the pan into the oven. Flip the sandwiches halfway through the cooking time. When cooking is complete, remove the pan from the oven. Divide the sandwiches among four plates and serve warm.

Nutrition: Calories 150 Carbs 34g Fiber 5g Protein 4g

Nutty Banana Bread

Serves: 8   Prep Time: 10 mins.   Cooking Time: 20 mins.

Ingredients

3 bananas, peeled and sliced 2/3 cup sugar 1 teaspoon of ground cinnamon

1 teaspoon of salt 1 1/3 cups of flour

1 teaspoon of baking soda

1 teaspoon of baking powder ½ cup of milk

½ cup of olive oil

Directions

Cream together all the wet ingredients in a bowl. Strain together all the dry ingredients in another bowl. Mix well to form a dough and place in the loaf pan. Place the loaf pan in the cooking tray. Set the Instant Vortex on Air fryer to 335 degrees F for 20 minutes. Insert the cooking tray in the Vortex when it displays "Add Food". Remove from the oven when cooking time is complete. Serve warm.

Nutrition: Calories: 295   Protein: 3.1g Carbs: 44g   Fat: 13.3g

Cauliflower Rice

Servings: 2   Preparation Time: 10 minutes Cooking Time: 22 minutes

Ingredients:

1 cauliflower head, cut into florets 1/2 tsp cumin 1/2 tsp chili powder

6 onion spring, chopped 2 jalapenos, chopped

4 tbsp olive oil

1 zucchini, trimmed and cut into cubes 1/2 tsp paprika 1/2 tsp garlic powder

1/2 tsp cayenne pepper 1/2 tsp pepper

1/2 tsp salt

Directions:

Preheat the air fryer to 370 F, add cauliflower florets into the food processor and process until it looks like rice. Transfer cauliflower rice into the air fryer baking pan and Drizzle with half oil, place pan in the air fryer and cook for 12 minutes, stir halfway through.

Heat the remaining oil in a small pan over medium heat, add zucchini and cook for 5-8 minutes. Add onion and jalapenos and cook for 5 minutes, add spices and stir well. Set aside. Add cauliflower rice in the zucchini mixture and stir well. Serve and enjoy.

Nutrition: Calories 254 Fat 28 g Carbs 12.3 g Protein 4.3 g

Bacon Cup

Serves: 6   Prep Time: 10 mins.   Cooking Time: 15 mins.

Ingredients

6 bacon slices

6 bread slices

1 scallion, chopped

2 teaspoons of almond extract

2 cups of pecans, finely chopped

3 tablespoons of green bell pepper, seeded and chopped 6 eggs

2 tablespoons of low-fat mayonnaise 2 cups of confectioners' sugar Directions

Place the bacon slices at the bottom of 6 greased muffin tins. Cut the bread slices into round shapes and place over the bacon slices. Top with scallion, bell pepper, and mayonnaise. Crack eggs over the top and arrange the muffin tins in the cooking tray. Set the Instant Vortex on Air fryer to 375 degrees F for 15 minutes. Insert the cooking tray in the Vortex when it displays "Add Food". Remove from the oven when cooking time is complete. Serve warm.

Nutrition: Calories: 260Protein: 16.1g Carbs: 6.9g Fat: 18g

Cheesy Tater Tot Breakfast Bake Casserole

Servings: 4   Preparation Time: 5 minutes Cooking Time: 20 minutes

Ingredients:

4 eggs

1 cup milk

1 teaspoon onion powder Salt, to taste

Pepper, to taste Cooking oil

12 ounces ground chicken sausage 1-pound frozen tater tots

¾ cup shredded Cheddar cheese

Directions:

In a medium bowl, whisk the eggs. Add the milk, onion powder, and salt and pepper to taste. Stir to combine, spray a skillet with cooking oil and set over medium-high heat. Add the ground sausage. Using a spatula or spoon, break the sausage into smaller pieces. Cook for 3 to 4 minutes, until the sausage is brown. Remove from heat and set aside. Spray a casserole with cooking oil. Make sure to cover the bottom and sides of the casserole, place the tater tots in the oven.

Cook for 6 minutes. Open the air fryer and shake the pan, then add the egg mixture and cooked sausage. Cook for an additional 6 minutes. Open the air fryer and sprinkle the cheese over the tater tot bake. Cook for an additional 2 to 3 minutes. Cool before serving.

Nutrition: Calories 518 Fat 30g Carbs 31g Protein 30g

Flavorful Protein Rich Breakfast

Serves: 4   Prep Time: 10 mins.   Cooking Time: 23 mins.

Ingredients:

7- ounces of ham, sliced 4 teaspoons of milk

1 tablespoon of olive oil

1 tablespoon of unsalted butter, melted 1 pound of fresh baby spinach

4 eggs

Salt and black pepper, to taste

Directions:

Put olive oil and spinach in a skillet on medium heat. Sauté for about 3 minutes and drain the spinach completely. Transfer this spinach into the ramekins and layer with ham slices. Crack 1 egg into each ramekin over ham slices and pour in the milk. Sprinkle with salt and black pepper and place in the cooking tray. Set the Instant Vortex on Air fryer to 355 degrees F for 20 minutes. Insert the cooking tray in the Vortex when it displays "Add Food". Remove from the oven when cooking time is complete. Serve hot.

Nutrition: Calories: 228   Protein: 17.2g Carbs: 6.6g   Fat: 15.8g

Breakfast Scramble Casserole

Servings: 4   Preparation Time: 20 minutes Cooking Time: 10 minutes

Ingredients:

6 slices bacon

6 eggs Salt Pepper Cooking oil

½ cup chopped red bell pepper ½ cup chopped green bell pepper ½ cup chopped onion

¾ cup shredded Cheddar cheese

Directions:

In a pan, over medium-high heat, cook the bacon, 5 to 7 minutes, flipping to evenly crisp. Dry out on paper towels, crumble, and set aside. In a medium bowl, whisk the eggs. Add salt and pepper to taste. Spray a barrel pan with cooking oil. Make sure to cover the bottom and sides of the pan. Add the beaten eggs, crumbled bacon, red bell pepper, green bell pepper, and onion to the pan, place the pan in the air fryer. Cook for 6 minutes Open the air fryer and sprinkle the cheese over the casserole. If you want cook for an additional 2 minutes. Cool before serving.

Nutrition: Calories 348 Fat 26g Carbs 4g Protein 25g

Egg In A Bread Basket

Serves: 2   Prep Time: 10 mins.   Cooking Time: 10 mins.

Ingredients:

2 bread slices

2 eggs

½ tablespoon of olive oil

1/8 teaspoon of maple syrup

1/8 teaspoon of balsamic vinegar ¼ teaspoon of fresh parsley, chopped Salt and black pepper, to taste

2 tablespoons of mayonnaise 1 bacon slice, chopped

4 tomato slices

1 tablespoon of Mozzarella cheese, shredded

Directions:

Grease 2 ramekins and arrange 1 bread slice in each ramekin. Add tomato and bacon slices and sprinkle with the Mozzarella cheese.

Crack 1 egg into each ramekin and pour in the balsamic vinegar and maple syrup. Sprinkle with parsley, salt and black pepper and place in the cooking tray. Set the Instant Vortex on Air fryer to 325 degrees F for 10 minutes. Insert the cooking tray in the Vortex when it displays "Add Food". Remove from the oven when cooking time is complete. Top with mayonnaise and serve hot.

Nutrition: Calories: 245Protein: 12.8 g Carbs: 10.2g Fat: 17.1g

Radish Hash Browns

Servings: 4   Preparation Time: 10 minutes Cooking Time: 13 minutes

Ingredients:

1 lb. radishes, washed and cut off roots 1 tbsp olive oil

1/2 tsp paprika

1/2 tsp onion powder 1/2 tsp garlic powder 1 medium onion

1/4 tsp pepper 3/4 tsp sea salt Directions:

Slice onion and radishes using a mandolin slicer, add sliced onion and radishes in a large mixing bowl and toss with olive oil. Transfer onion and radish slices in air fryer basket and cook at 360 F for 8 minutes Shake basket twice, return onion and radish slices in a mixing bowl and toss with seasonings. Again, cook onion and radish slices in air fryer basket for 5 minutes at 400 F. Shake the basket halfway through. Serve and enjoy.

Nutrition: Calories 62 Fat 3.7 g Carbs 7.1 g Protein 1.2 g

Delicious Tofu And Mushroom Omelet

Serves: 2   Prep Time: 10 mins.   Cooking Time: 25 mins.

Ingredients:

2 tablespoons of milk

2 teaspoons of canola oil

8- ounces of silken tofu, pressed and sliced 3½ ounces of fresh mushrooms, sliced

3 eggs, beaten

1 garlic clove, minced

Salt and black pepper, to taste

Directions:

Set the Instant Vortex on Air fryer to 360 degrees F for 25 minutes. Sauté garlic and onion in the canola oil for about 3 minutes in a pan. Fold in the tofu, mushrooms, salt, and black pepper. Stir well and pour into the cooking tray. Top with the beaten eggs and insert the cooking tray in the Vortex when it displays "Add Food". Remove from the oven when cooking time is complete. Serve hot.

Nutrition: Calories: 224Protein: 17.9g Carbs: 6.6g Fat: 14.5g

Asparagus Frittata

Servings: 4   Preparation Time: 10 minutes Cooking Time: 10 minutes

Ingredients:

6 eggs

3 mushrooms, sliced

10 asparagus, chopped 1/4 cup half and half

2 tsp butter, melted

1 cup mozzarella cheese, shredded 1 tsp pepper

1 tsp salt

Directions:

Toss mushrooms and asparagus with melted butter and add into the air fryer basket. Cook mushrooms and asparagus at 350 F for 5 minutes Shake basket twice, meanwhile, in a bowl, whisk together eggs, half and half, pepper, and salt. Transfer cook mushrooms and asparagus into the air fryer baking dish. Pour egg mixture over mushrooms and asparagus. Place dish in the air fryer and cook at 350 F for 5 minutes or until eggs are set. Slice and serve.

Nutrition: Calories 211 Fat 13 g Carbs 4 g Protein 16 g

Special Eggs, Mushroom And Tomato Scramble

Serves: 4   Prep Time: 15 mins.   Cooking Time: 11 mins.

Ingredients:

½ cup of mushrooms, sliced

1 tablespoon of chives, chopped ¾ cup of milk 4 eggs

8 grape tomatoes, halved

Salt and black pepper, to taste

Directions:

Set the Instant Vortex on Air fryer to 360 degrees F for 6 minutes. Whip eggs with milk, salt, and black pepper in a bowl. Pour the egg mixture into the cooking tray. Insert the cooking tray in the Vortex when it displays "Add Food". Remove from the oven when cooking time is complete. Stir in the mushrooms, chives, and grape tomatoes. Cook in the vortex again for about 5 minutes and serve hot.

Nutrition: Calories: 132Protein: 9.5g Carbs: 12.5g
Fat: 5.8g

Yummy Ham, Spinach, And Egg In A Cup

Serves: 4   Prep Time: 10 mins.   Cooking Time: 8 mins.

Ingredients:

4 eggs

4 thick slices of deli ham

4 tablespoons of spinach, chopped Black pepper, to taste 4 tablespoons of cheddar cheese, shredded

Directions:

Grease 4 muffin tins and put the ham slices in it. Press the muffin tins into cups gently. Stir in the spinach and cheddar cheese. Top with the eggs and keep aside. Set the Instant Vortex on Air fryer to 375 degrees F for 8 minutes. Insert the cooking tray in the Vortex when it displays "Add Food". Remove from the oven when cooking time is complete and egg yolk is done to desired firmness.

Nutrition: Calories: 228   Protein: 17.2g
Carbs: 6.6g   Fat: 15.6g

Mini Brown Rice Quiches

Serves 6   Prep time: 10 minutes Cook time: 14 minutes

Ingredients:

4 ounces (113 g) diced green chilies 3 cups cooked brown rice

1 cup shredded reduced-fat Cheddar cheese, divided ½ cup egg whites

⅓ cup fat-free milk

¼ cup diced pimiento

½ teaspoon cumin

1 small eggplant, cubed

1 bunch fresh cilantro, finely chopped Cooking spray

Directions:

Spritz a 12-cup muffin pan with cooking spray, In a large bowl, stir together all the ingredients, except for ½ cup of the cheese. Scoop the mixture evenly into the muffin cups and sprinkle the remaining ½ cup of the cheese on top, select Bake. Set temperature to 400°F (205°C) and set time to 14 minutes. Select Start to begin preheating. Once the unit has preheated, slide the pan into the oven, when cooking is complete, remove the pan and check the quiches. They should be set. Carefully transfer the quiches to a platter and serve immediately.

Nutrition: Calories: 245Protein: 12.8 g Carbs: 10.2g Fat: 17.1g

Glazed Strawberry Toast

Servings 4 toasts   Prep time: 5 minutes Cook time: 8 minutes

Ingredients:

4 slices bread, ½-inch thick 1 cup sliced strawberries

1 teaspoon sugar Cooking spray Directions:

On a clean work surface, lay the bread slices and spritz one side of each slice of bread with cooking spray, place the bread slices in a perforated pan, sprayed side down. Top with the strawberries and a sprinkle of sugar. Select Air Fry, set temperature to 375°F (190°C), and set time to 8 minutes. Select Start to begin preheating, once preheated, slide the pan into the oven. When cooking is complete, the toast should be well browned on each side. Remove from the oven to a plate and serve.

Nutrition: Calories: 397Protein: 27.3g Carbs: 17.8g Fat: 26.2g

Ham Omelet

Serves: 2   Prep Time: 10 mins.   Cooking Time: 30 mins.

Ingredients:

1 onion, chopped

2 tablespoons of cheddar cheese 4 small tomatoes, chopped

2 ham slices

Salt and black pepper, to taste 4 eggs

Directions:

Put onion and ham on medium heat in a nonstick skillet. Sauté for about 5 minutes and place in the cooking tray along with the tomatoes. Whip eggs with salt and black pepper in a bowl. Drizzle the egg mixture in the cooking tray and top with the cheddar cheese. Set the Instant Vortex on Air fryer to 390 degrees F for 10 minutes.

Insert the cooking tray in the Vortex when it displays "Add Food". Remove from the oven when cooking time is complete.

Serve warm with toasts.

Nutrition: Calories: 255Protein: 19.7g Carbs: 14.1g Fat: 13.9g

Turkey Breakfast Sausage Patties

Serves 4   Prep time: 5 minutes Cook time: 10 minutes

Ingredients:

1 tablespoon chopped fresh thyme

1 tablespoon chopped fresh sage

1 teaspoon crushed fennel seeds

¾ teaspoon smoked paprika

½ teaspoon onion powder

½ teaspoon garlic powder

⅛ teaspoon crushed red pepper flakes

⅛ teaspoon freshly ground black pepper 1 pound (454 g) 93% lean ground turkey

½ cup finely minced sweet apple

salt

Directions:

Thoroughly combine the thyme, sage, salt, fennel seeds, paprika, onion powder, garlic powder, red pepper flakes, and black pepper in a medium bowl, add the ground turkey and apple and stir until well incorporated. Divide the mixture into 8 equal portions and shape into patties with your hands, each about ¼ inch thick and 3 inches in diameter. Place the patties in a perforated pan in a single layer, select Air Fry, set temperature to 400°F (205°C), and set time to 10 minutes. Select Start to begin preheating. Once preheated, slide the pan into the oven. Flip the patties halfway through the cooking time, when cooking is complete, the patties should be nicely browned and cooked through. Remove from the oven to a plate and serve warm.

Nutrition: Calories: 397Protein: 27.3g Carbs: 17.8g Fat: 26.2g

Tasty Cream Bread

Serves: 12   Prep Time: 20 mins.   Cooking Time: 15 mins.

Ingredients:

2 tablespoons of milk powder

¾ cup of whipping cream 1 teaspoon of salt

1 cup of milk 1 large egg

4½ cups of bread flour

½ cup of all-purpose flour ¼ cup of fine sugar 3 teaspoons of dry yeast

Directions:

Cream together all the wet ingredients in a bowl. Strain together all the dry ingredients in another bowl. Combine the two mixtures to form a dough and divide it into 4 pieces. Spread each piece. into a rectangle and roll tightly like a Swiss roll. Place the rolls in the cooking tray. Set the Instant Vortex on Air fryer to 375 degrees F for 15 minutes. Insert the cooking tray in the Vortex when it displays "Add Food". Remove from the oven when cooking time is complete. Cut into preferred size slices and serve immediately.

Nutrition: Calories: 215   Protein: 6.5g Carbs: 36.9g   Fat: 3.1g

Cheese Soufflés

Servings: 8   Preparation Time: 10 minutes Cooking Time: 6 minutes

Ingredients:

6 large eggs, separated
3/4 cup heavy cream
1/4 tsp cayenne pepper
1/2 tsp xanthan gum
1/2 tsp pepper

1/4 tsp cream of tartar
2 tbsp chives, chopped

2 cups cheddar cheese, shredded
1 tsp salt

Directions:

Preheat the air fryer to 325 F. spray eight ramekins with cooking spray. Set aside. In a bowl, whisk together almond flour, cayenne pepper, pepper, salt, and xanthan gum, slowly add heavy cream and mix to combine. Whisk in egg yolks, chives, and cheese until well combined, In a large bowl, add egg whites and cream of tartar and beat until stiff peaks form. Fold egg white mixture into the almond flour mixture until combined, pour mixture into the prepared ramekins. Divide ramekins in batches. Place the first batch of ramekins into the air fryer basket, cook soufflé for 20 minutes. Serve and enjoy.

Nutrition: Calories 210 Fat 16 g Carbs 1 g Protein 12 g

CHURROS FINGERS WITH CHOCOLATE DIPPING SAUCE

Servings 4 | Prep Time 8 mins | Cooking Time 15 mins

5 tsp butter, unsalted

1 tsp sugar

1-cup water

1-cup flour, all-purpose type

2 medium eggs

1/8 tsp salt

1/8 tsp nutmeg

1-cup dark chocolate, chopped into small cubes

In a saucepan, heat up water, butter and sugar. Make sure to put it on high until the sugar is melted completely.

Stir the butter until it melts. Add the flour and stir quickly to make a paste.

Put the heat to low. It will take longer and it will be hot, but you can reduce the heat. Stir the food a lot while it is cooking until it starts to come away from the sides of your pan. It should be firm when you are done

Remove the mixture from heat and let it cool for ten minutes. Then beat in the eggs and salt.

Mixture should be smooth and glossy.

Transfer the mixture from the bowl to a pastry bag with a star shaped nozzle. Then, pipe the mixture into any shape you want on your baking pan.

Place the pan in position 2 and set oven to air fry on 390°F for 6 minutes.

Cook until crisp and golden brown. Repeat with remaining batter.

Put chocolate, water and sugar in a double boiler. Let them sit until they have completely melted. Stir it occasionally while you wait.

When the mixture is melted, stir in butter. Keep cooking until it's all mixed together. Serve with churros.

Calories 645 | Fat 37g | Carbs 68g | Protein 12g

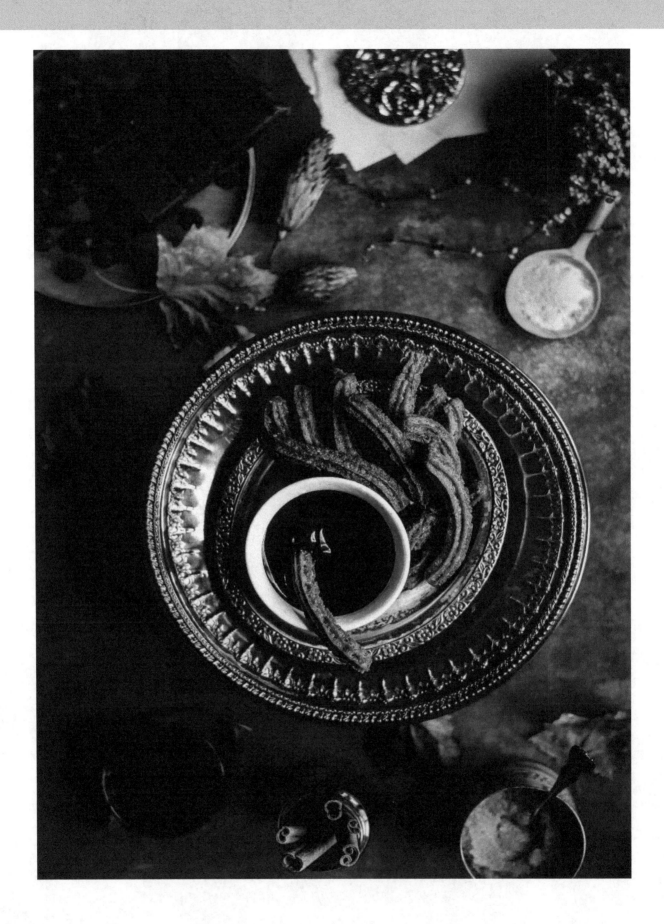

BISCUITS DONUTS

Serves 4 | Prep Time 7 mins | Cooking Time 5 mins.

Coconut oil

can of biscuit dough, pre-made

1/2 cup of white sugar

1/2 cup of powdered sugar

tablespoons of melted butter

2 teaspoons of cinnamon

     Set the Instant Vortex on Air fryer to 350 degrees F for 5 minutes.

     Cut the dough with a biscuit cutter. Then brush the cooking tray with coconut oil.

     Place biscuits on it when a screen says "Add Food."

When the oven says "Turn Food" turn the pan. Cook for the time that is on the oven. When it is done, then pour in melted butter and cover with your topping. Serve while warm!

Calories 305 | Protein 8.9g | Carbs 27g | Fat 33.2g

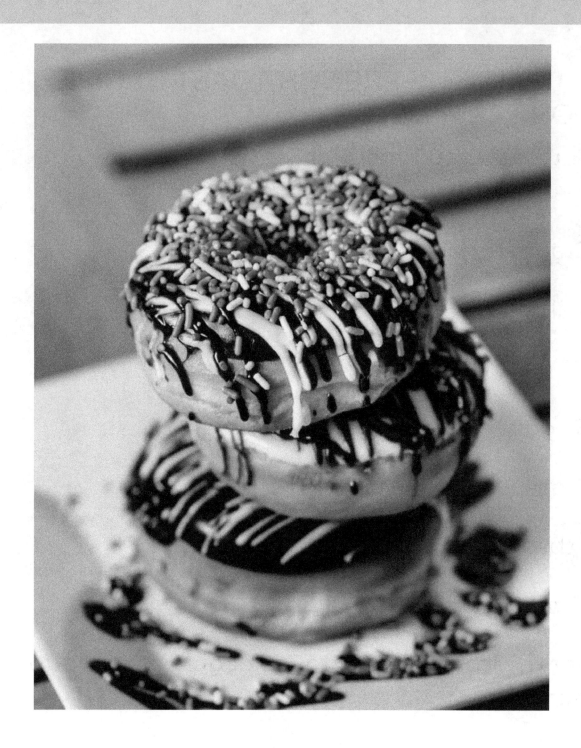

A DELICIOUS FRENCH TOAST RECIPE FOR YOUR LOVER

Serves: 2 Prep Time: 12 mins. Cooking Time: 7 mins.

Cranberry jam

4 slices of bread

1/6 cup skimmed milk

3 eggs

1 teaspoon ground cinnamon

1 tbsp brown sugar

Salt

Set the Instant Vortex to 375 degrees on Bake for 4 minutes.

In a low and wide dish break the eggs, add a pinch of salt and begin to beat them, without stopping, add the milk and then add the cinnamon.

Mix again and set aside for a moment.

Preheat your Instant Vortex to 350' F on Bake

Soak bread in mixture and place on rack.

Let the rack sit over the plate to drain a little.

Cook for 3 minutes and then flip. Cook for 5 minutes total. You may need to add a few minutes to get them golden brown.

Serve hot with cranberry jam and a cup of tea. and serve with tea. Calories: 248 | Protein: 7.5g | Carbs: 27.2g | Fat:2.3g

Functions of Vortex Air Fryer Oven

The Vortex Air Fryer Oven comes with a touch screen LED display and various functions that are used during the

The vortex air fryer has a touch panel that is digital. You can use it to cook your food automatically or manually.

7 Different Smart Programs/Function Modes

The smart programs are automated. They are programmed to do things like set the time or temperature. When you use these functions you never need to set them yourself. When the oven goes into standby mode, it will display "OFF". These smart programs are:

1. Air Fry

2. Broil

3. Roast

4. Bake

5. Dehydrate

6.   Reheat

Start

The Start button is used to start the cooking process.

 Cancel

As the name suggests, when you press cancel, it will stop your cooking. When you press cancel, it will stop your cooking and then go on standby mode.

Light

The Light button is used to turn ON and OFF the oven light. After 5 minutes of time oven light turn OFF automatically.

(+ / -) Temperature Controls (Temp)

The (+) button is used to make the temperature higher and the (-) button is used to make the temperature lower.

(+ / -) Time

You can use the (+ / -) time button to change the cooking time on your stove. To increase cooking time, touch and hold "+". To decrease cooking time, touch and hold "-".

Rotate

When you start the cooking process, the Rotate button will turn on. You just need to touch it once more to stop the rotisserie. This button is only available when you choose Air Fry or Roast in the cooking process. When the key turns blue, then it means that you can use it.

CPSIA information can be obtained
at www.ICGtesting.com
Printed in the USA
BVHW010316160621
609629BV00016B/1686

9 781802 114805